50 TOP KETOGENIC RECIPES

Quick and Easy Keto Diet Recipes for Weight Loss and Optimum Health

GEMMA GREEN

Book

5

CONTENTS

"I love everything about Emma's connection to weight loss and health."

Hi, my name is Nat Lee, and I've spent most of my life looking pretty good and feeling great. That was up until I started eating on the run and allowing my busy life as a mom to take hold of me. While working too.

In truth, I knew I should eat great food, but time constraints and "motherly craziness" got the better of me. I made sure my son ate well. But I didn't, which was silly, really. Parenting is one of those things that just takes over your life, I suppose. So, anyway, I kinda ate loads of stuff I shouldn't, and drank sodas and milkshakes an awful lot. Chocolate and takeout became my best friend, and I became overweight, by anyone's standards. No one really told me I looked bad, I mean, most people aren't that obvious. But when I was diagnosed with a severe illness and bedridden for four years, it became time to do something to help my recovery. I made the change as soon as I could.

Since reading Emma's books, I've lost 18.5 kg (which is 40 amazing pounds). And I've managed to keep it off by following her wonderful advice, and by using her awesome, easy-to-do recipes. I live relatively simply, but her guide to nutrition and her tips and tricks have helped me a bucket load. Thank you, Emma, you've literally changed my life!

MY STORY

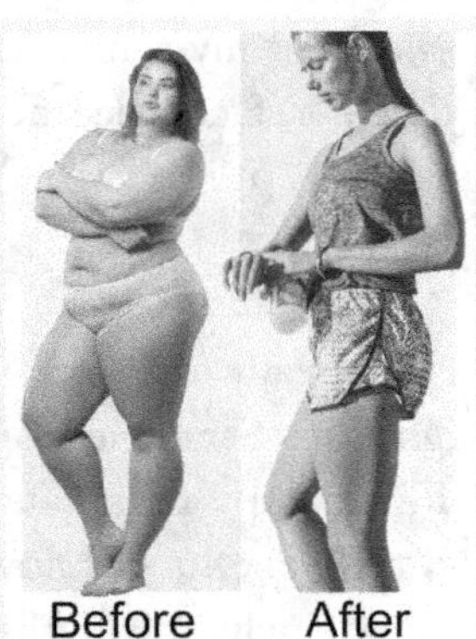

Hi, and thank you so much for joining me here! I absolutely love that you've come to share your time with me. My name is Emma Green and I have lost over 100 pounds, through the use of living healthily and staying positive (as a combining effort).

I know that if you are looking to lose weight, you've definitely come to the right place. I am absolutely sure that when you combine great nutrition with positivity and maintaining a stress-free environment as much as you can, then you'll be able to get where you are going. And, I want you to do that faster, safer, and with your health always at the forefront of your mind.

I want to tell you a bit about me. After a time, I got diagnosed with arthritis. I think the arthritis was diagnosed between 27 and 28 years of age, from memory. It was a major pain in the neck, quite literally. I had excessive knee pain and standing for long periods was excruciating, some days. It took so long sometimes, to do even little things. The pain was unbearable in my back as well. I also loved to cook, but everything ached so much at times, that even that was hard to do. The news literally shocked me when I heard it. The experience of it sucked more than I can put into words. I was in pain most days, more than not. A symptom of my obesity, so I was told. The pressure in the body from taking up the excess load became a real nightmare. I had to make a change. For my health's sake, and my sanity. I researched all the best tips, tricks, and ways to do it. In fact, I learned to do it in safety and efficiency. I lost the weight and kept it off.

Please know, if you haven't already read my title, "How I Lost 100 Pounds! My Personal Weight Loss Strategies for Optimum Happiness," make sure you get your FREE copy today. Inside you'll learn exactly how I lost my weight, and the benefits of knowing the must-do nutrition, and other amazing secrets including myths, water weight, cellulite prevention and removal, the only exercise you really need, the ancient and easy technique to help slim you quickly, how to balance meals, and much, much more! I hope you love it. It's my very special gift to you!

So, how do you keep positive and lose weight at the same time? I have a few great ideas. My favorites are: goal planning, meditation, yoga, walking, light aerobics, spending time with friends and family, watching funny movies, cooking, art, listening to music, and dancing (in my room so no one else can see!)

Take a moment now and think about what makes you happy... and what your goals are, both for the short term and the long term... now how will you achieve the happy part - and the goals? What do you need to do to make it work? Write that down, too. Now, after you've worked that out, I want you to plan it out on paper. Start with monthly, then break it down to weekly, and then break it down to daily. It might take some time, but you'll be glad you did.

If you have a plan, then you can work toward your goal/s. Without one it's really hard to know why you are doing what you are, and the time-frames and routes you need to take to do so. For example, if I say, "I want to lose weight," that statement is great. But if I don't have a plan of action, then I can't really follow through on it, definitively. And that's because I need to know how to get there. So, if I make a plan (for meal types, meal times, exercise types, exercise times, relaxation time, a no-go foods list, time needed for preparation of meals, time needed for workouts etc.) then I can really know exactly what's needed. Breaking it into chunks (daily) will allow me to succeed, because I'll only have to deal with those "actions" or "timetables" daily. It's easy when you plan.

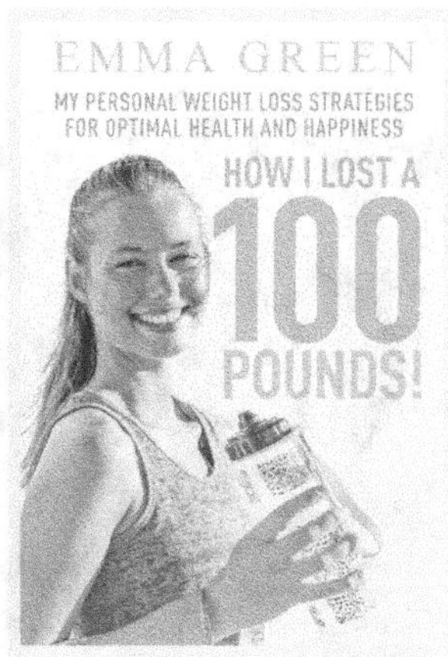

Btw check out "How i lost a 100 pounds" if you haven't already, its got loads of value and its completely FREE :)

FREE GIFTS!

Here are 3 bonus books I want to gift you for coming and reading this title! Sign up to my newsletter and you will receive:

Weight Loss Myths - 9 myths that you are mostly likely doing right now that are totally pointless and are a waste of time toward your weight loss goals.

How to Lose Weight Fast – A 10 day plan I personally put together to make that weight literally melt before your eyes (it worked for me!)

And... Weight Loss Secrets - Secrets the main stream media and health industry never talk about because (let's be honest) things that work don't make them money!

Click here to sign up! or for paperback versions grab it through the ebook completely FREE!

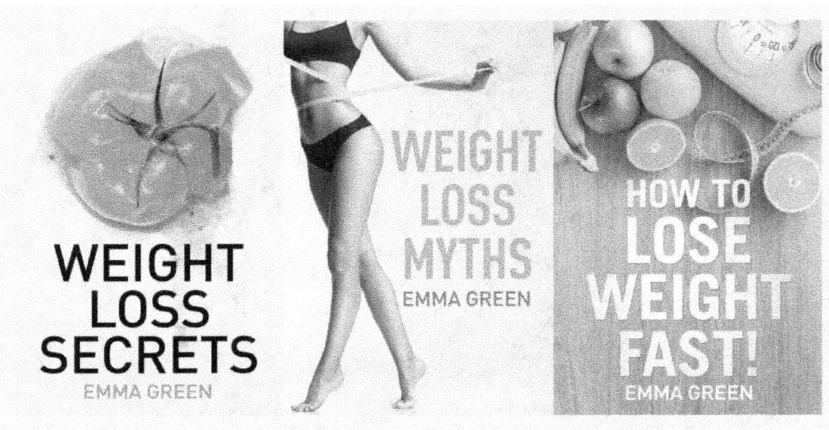

Chapter One

THE HEALTH ISSUES FROM A CONVENTIONAL US-BASED DIET

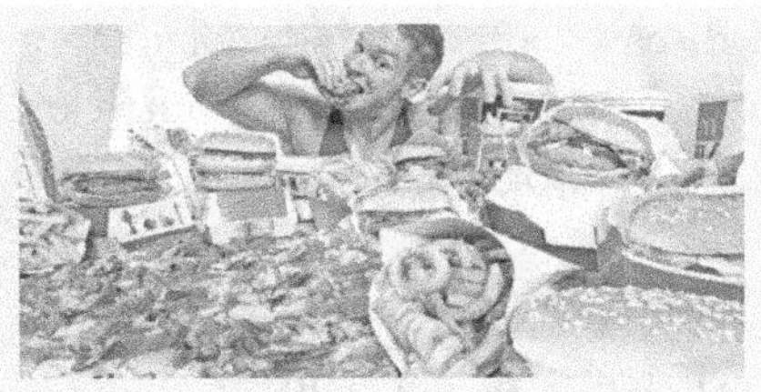

Statistically speaking, over 117 million adults have a health issue or disease that can be combated through simple lifestyle changes. And ultimately, nutrition is a big part of that change. That is a HUGE statistic, and one that's literally changing and shortening the longevity of people living in America today, unfortunately.

I want you to know that YOU can do this! Losing weight is possible when you know how. So, let's take a look at some of the sad, mind-blowing statistics that will keep us motivated toward our end goal. Losing weight isn't just for "looks" but it is, more importantly, for our overall health.

Shocking Statistics:

- Obesity rates now exceed 35 % in five states, 30% in 25 states, and 25% in 46 states. With West Virginia leading at 37.7% in 2017.
- 36.5 % of U.S. adults are obese.
- Obesity-related conditions include stroke, type 2 diabetes, heart disease, and certain cancers.
- The annual cost of obesity in the U.S. is over $147 billion each year.
- Medical costs for people with obesity are annually $1400 more per annum than for individuals within a normal weight range.

Unfortunately, these statistics are growing, and have been climbing for children, too. The diseases affecting us today can actually be negated and minimized through the use of great nutrition, exercise, and by changing other lifestyle factors that can cause stress.

I believe that knowledge is power, and we can share this knowledge with our family, friends and our children as well. And then, over time, we can change the world. Let's do that, starting with you and me...

Chapter Two

THE BENEFITS OF KETO FOR WEIGHT LOSS

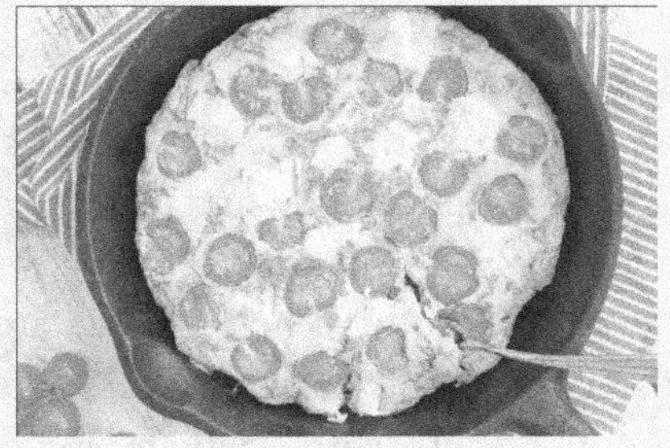

One summer afternoon, I had been cooking with mum. We were trying a stir-fry recipe that we saw in an Asian cookbook. While she finished the preparation and began cooking, I spent a few minutes looking for recipes online. "Ketogenic recipes for weight loss" came up, and I thought, wow, I think I've heard some great stuff about that.

I flicked through and looked at the recipes. Most of them were with foods I loved, and with relatively easy-to-do instructions. I couldn't believe I could eat "like that" and lose weight as well. So, I researched it more and found out why! Even my mom was shocked at how good the recipes were. She said, "They'll be yummy too!" And so, I never looked back after that. It was the start of something beautiful. The new, fat-burning version of me!

The ketogenic diet consists of consuming a low amount of carbohydrates and replacing them with fats and oils. After a short time of reducing these carbs, your body ends up in what is called a "state of ketosis." It is while in this state that the body becomes highly efficient at burning fat.

Keto Science

Ketosis happens on a daily basis, yet usually on a much smaller scale if that's not the focus. When we consume carbs, these become converted to glucose, which is the fuel for the brain and the body. When we have an excess of glucose, this gets stored (as fat). On a keto diet, as fewer carbohydrates are consumed, the body enters ketosis and looks to the fat deposits for more energy. Ketones are created by the liver and used as the energy source for the body. When the fats are broken down by the liver, fatty acids and glycerol are released. The fatty acids become broken down to produce acetoacetate which is converted into beta-hydroxybutyrate (which the brain loves), and into acetone which can be turned into glucose (although the majority of that is excreted as waste).

Studies show us that the body operates more efficiently using these ketones than glucose. The basis of the diet was first discovered by Dr. Henry Rawle Geyelin (1921) who found that while a person was in a state of fasting, their glucose levels dropped. However, at the same time, their ketone levels increased, which in turn, placed less stress on the brain.

Keto Diet and Weight Loss

The keto diet is so good at helping you to lose weight that you are in a position to not have to focus on the calories you consume on a daily basis. You also have the benefit of feeling more satisfied at meal times, so you will have less need to eat in-between meals.

Various studies show us that the keto diet is far superior to other diets for losing weight. Results were compared in a study in England. The Diabetes UK diet was followed by some participants while the Keto diet was followed by others. At the end of the study, it showed the participants on the Keto diet had lost up to three times more weight in a period of just three months.

Food Types to Eat

Food types you should focus your attention on eating while you are on the keto diet are as listed. Please know that this list is not comprehensive, yet it gives a good oversight of what you can consume:

Low Carb Vegetables: Most varieties of green vegetables along with tomatoes, peppers, onions and many others.

Meat: Red meat, bacon, sausages, steak, turkey, and chicken.

Fatty Fish: Mackerel, tuna, salmon, trout and others.

Butter and Cream: These should come from grass fed (organic) cows, where possible.

Cheeses: Mozzarella, cream cheese, goat, and cheddar (as long as they are not overly-processed).

Healthy Oils: Avocado oil, extra virgin olive oil, and coconut oil.

Nuts and Seeds: Chia seeds, pumpkin seeds, flaxseeds, walnuts, and almonds.

Eggs: These should be free-range where possible.

Avocado: These can be consumed as they are, or as fresh guacamole.

Condiments: Sea salt and pepper along with most herbs and spices can be used.

Other Important Factors

The keto diet was initially created as a treatment for epilepsy in children. It has to be said; it excelled much better than many man-made drugs at that time. It should be noted, however, that there can be **consequences for children that follow the keto diet**. Making sure that children have a wide range of vitamins and nutrients is always paramount for growth and development. There is also the possibility that children could become affected by kidney stones, or (depending on their age) have stunted growth. Additionally, the risk of bone fractures is increased as the growth factor 1 hormone production is reduced.

You might be wondering how long you should follow the ketogenic diet for. It can take anywhere between a couple of days to a little over a week for the body to enter a state of ketosis. There is also no hard evidence that states any length of time a person can stay on the keto diet for, but current recommendations give a period of three months maximum, before taking a break from following it, "religiously." Some individuals continue to follow the keto diet for a few days per week, and on the other days they revert to a regular, healthy, eating plan. Safe dieting is always recommended.

Now, let's get to the recipes, I'm so excited to share them with you!

Chapter Three

KETOGENIC BREAKFAST RECIPES

Recipe 1

MARVELOUS MINI-KETO QUICHES

"Great with friends... they'll love it!"

Ingredients

- 14 eggs
- 3 plum tomatoes, diced
- 2/3 of a cup of mozzarella cheese torn into bite-size pieces
- 1/3 of a cup of cheddar cheese, grated
- 1/3 of a cup of white onion, diced finely
- 1/3 of a cup of pickled jalapenos, sliced
- 2/3 of a cup of salami, diced
- 1/3 of a cup of heavy cream
- 1 pinch of sea salt and black pepper, to taste

Instructions

- Preheat oven to 160 degrees C and lightly grease a muffin tin. Half fill any muffin trays with water.
- In a mixing bowl, beat the eggs.
- Add to the mixing bowl all remaining ingredients and mix well, then season with salt and pepper.
- Divide the batter into the muffin tins equally, and bake for around 25 minutes.
- Can be stored in the refrigerator and reheated before eating.

KETO PEANUT MUFFINS: RECIPE 2

Ingredients

- 1 cup of almond flour, sifted
- 3 tablespoons of honey
- 1 teaspoon of baking powder
- 1 pinch of sea salt
- 1/3 of a cup of peanut butter
- 1/3 of a cup of almond milk
- 2 eggs

Instructions

- Preheat oven to 180 degrees C.
- Take a large mixing bowl and add all of the dry ingredients and mix well.
- Add the almond milk and the peanut butter, then stir until well combined.
- Add 1 egg at a time and incorporate each fully.
- Spray the muffin tins with non-stick spray.
- Divide batter into muffin tins to 3/4 full.
- Bake for around 15 to 20 minutes.

MOZZARELLA AND PEPPERONI-OMELET PIZZA: RECIPE 3

Ingredients

- 3 large eggs
- 2 strips of bacon
- 1 tablespoon of heavy cream
- 1/2 an oz. of pepperoni slices
- 1/2 of a cup of shredded mozzarella, bite size pieces
- salt and pepper, to taste
- 1 tablespoon of fresh basil, chopped

Instructions

- Heat a medium sized skillet over medium heat, add the bacon slices and cook until your desired crispiness. Remove and set aside.
- In a mixing bowl, beat the eggs. Add the heavy cream and then combine and pour into the skillet. Cook until almost done.
- Add pepperoni slices to one half of the cooked egg, and then sprinkle with mozzarella pieces.
- Season with salt and pepper, then sprinkle with basil.
- Fold the omelet over, and then cook for a further 1 to 2 minutes, turning once to cook through.
- Serve warm with bacon slices.

KETO-POWERED BREAKFAST SMOOTHIE: RECIPE 4

"This one gives you loads of energy!"

Ingredients

- 1 and a 1/2 cup of almond milk
- 1 oz. of spinach
- 1/2 a medium avocado, seeded and peeled

- 1 tablespoon of coconut oil
- powered sweetener to taste (optional)
- 1 scoop of vanilla-flavored protein powder

Instructions

- Add all the ingredients in a blender.
- Blend on high until everything is smooth and creamy.
- Scrape down the sides if anything sticks.

YUMMY SAUSAGE AND EGG WITH CHEESE: RECIPE 5

Ingredients

- 3 oz. of breakfast sausage
- 1 egg
- 1 tablespoon of olive oil
- 1 cheddar cheese slice
- chives or spring onion for garnish, chopped

Instructions

- Heat a small skillet over medium heat and add olive oil, cook sausage until no longer pink, and browned on all sides.
- In the same pan, cook the egg until the desired "doneness" is reached.
- Transfer to a serving plate and garnish with chives or green onion.

KETO-SPICED CHAI MICROWAVE CAKE: RECIPE 6

Ingredients

- 1 egg
- 2 tablespoons of butter, unsalted
- 2 tablespoons of almond flour

- 1 tablespoon of sweetener (optional, honey is great, to taste)
- 7 drops of liquid stevia
- 1/2 a teaspoon of baking powder
- 1/4 of a teaspoon of cinnamon
- 1/4 of a teaspoon of ginger
- 1/4 of a teaspoon of cloves
- 1/4 of a teaspoon of vanilla extract
- a sprinkle of cinnamon, to garnish
- 2 tablespoons of heavy cream

Instructions

- Mix all ingredients together in a large mug.
- Microwave on high for 70 seconds, approximately.
- Turn the mug upside down and lightly bang it against a plate or eat it directly from the mug.
- It should hold its form.
- Top with a little heavy cream and cinnamon.

WONDERFULLY-WARMING WINTER PORRIDGE: RECIPE 7

"Do this for winter as a snack too! I like to add extra cinnamon."

Ingredients

- 2 tablespoons of hemp seeds
- 1/4 of a cup of walnuts or pecans, chopped
- 1/4 of a cup of coconut, flaked
- 2 tablespoon of chia seeds
- 3/4 of a cup of almond milk, unsweetened
- 1/4 of a cup of coconut milk
- 1 tablespoon of sweetener (of choice) to taste (optional)

- 1/4 of a cup of almond butter, roasted
- 1 tablespoon of coconut oil
- ½ a teaspoon of ground turmeric
- 1 teaspoon of honey
- a good pinch of ground black pepper

Instructions

- Place a skillet over medium heat.
- Add the chopped walnuts/pecans, hemp seeds and the flaked coconut.
- Roast for 1 to 2 minutes and shake or toss to prevent burning. When cooked, place in a small bowl and set aside.
- In a small saucepan, heat the almond milk and coconut milk. As it comes to a low boil, remove from the heat, carefully. Add the coconut oil, turmeric powder, black pepper, almond butter, chia seeds, and the sweetener (to taste, optional).
- Stir until well combined and set aside. Stand for 5-10 minutes. Add half of the dry roasted mix from the bowl.
- Divide the porridge into two serving bowls. Top with the remaining dry roast mix.
- Drizzle with honey or cinnamon.

KETO CRÈME FRUITY: RECIPE 8

"Seasonal fruit can be added here, to taste."

Ingredients

- 1 tub of natural Greek yogurt
- 2 tablespoons of toasted almond flakes
- 2 tablespoons of toasted coconut flakes
- 6 tablespoons of fruit jelly, any flavor of choice can be used

Instructions

- Spoon 3 tablespoons of the fruit jelly into each serving bowl.
- Add half of the Greek yogurt into each serving bowl.
- Top with coconut flakes and almond flakes.

SPICED KETO PUMPKIN WAFFLES: RECIPE 9

Ingredients

- 2 eggs
- 2 tablespoons of butter, unsalted
- 2 tablespoons of heavy cream
- 1/2 a teaspoon of cinnamon powder
- 1/4 of a cup of pumpkin purée
- 1 scoop of whey protein powder, plain or vanilla
- 1 and a 1/2 tablespoons of coconut flour or almond flour
- 1 teaspoon of spiced pumpkin pie mix
- 1/4 of a teaspoon of baking soda
- 2 tablespoons of powdered sweetener (optional)
- 3 or 4 drops of vanilla extract

Instructions

- In a mixing bowl, add the eggs and whisk them together with the coconut oil, powdered sweetener (optional), and vanilla extract.
- Add the pureed pumpkin and heavy cream then whisk until you have a smooth batter.
- Add all the dry ingredients and beat together until well combined.
- Preheat waffle maker and cook mixture according to the waffle iron instructions.

ALL-DAY KETO BREAKFAST: RECIPE 10

Ingredients

- 2 eggs
- 6 bacon slices
- 1/2 a cup of mushrooms, fresh
- 1 avocado, peeled, pitted and sliced
- 1 tablespoon of butter, unsalted
- salt and black pepper, to taste

Instructions

- Place a skillet over medium heat, add half of butter, and then place the mushrooms top side down.
- Season with salt and pepper and cook for around 8 minutes.
- While the mushrooms are cooking, add butter to another small pan to fry the bacon and eggs to your desired liking.
- Transfer to serving plates along with the avocado slices as a garnish.

YUMMY BERRIES WITH COCONUT CREAM: RECIPE 11

"Use seasonally-available berries!"

Ingredients

- 4 cups of fresh berries, any choice, plain or mixed
- 5 leaves of fresh mint, and some more for garnish
- 1 can of full-fat coconut milk, chilled
- 2 teaspoons of vanilla extract
- 1 teaspoon of honey

Instructions

- Wash and drain the berries then divide into serving bowls.
- Chop the fresh mint finely and sprinkle over the berries.
- Open the can of chilled coconut milk. Use a spoon to scoop out the contents into a mixing bowl.
- Discard any juice or save it for another dish.
- Add the vanilla extract.
- Using a hand mixer, slowly beat the coconut cream. After around 1 minute just add the honey for sweetness (optional).
- Continue to mix until the coconut cream starts to become fluffy.
- Spoon over the berries and serve immediately.
- Garnish with the extra mint if required.

Chapter Four

KETOGENIC LUNCH RECIPES

Recipe 12: CHEDDAR AND HAM MAYO WRAPS

Ingredients

- 2 low carb wraps
- 4 to 5 tablespoons of mayonnaise
- 4 oz. of cheddar cheese, grated
- 4 oz. of sliced ham
- jalapenos or pickles, thinly sliced to taste
- sea salt and black pepper, to taste

Instructions

- Heat the skillet over medium heat, place wrap in a dry skillet and warm through for about 30 seconds.
- Take the warm wrap and spread the mayonnaise.
- Place ham slices on the wrap, and then sprinkle with the grated cheddar cheese.
- Add slices of pickle or jalapenos according to taste.
- Fold the ends inward and then roll tightly.

BLT MAYO WRAP WITH AVOCADO: RECIPE 13

"I like to add herbs like parsley and rosemary to this one!"

Ingredients

- 8 lettuce leaves
- 6 tablespoons of mayonnaise
- 12 strips of bacon
- 1 tomato, sliced thinly
- 1 avocado peeled, seeded, and thinly sliced
- 1 tablespoon of olive oil
- sea salt and black pepper, to taste

Instructions

- Heat a skillet over medium heat, add a dash of olive oil and cook the bacon to your liking.
- Wash and pat dry the lettuce leaves and then flatten slightly.
- Spread 1 tablespoon of mayonnaise onto each leaf.
- Season with salt and black pepper.
- Add 2 slices of bacon to each lettuce leaf.
- Divide the avocado slices and sliced tomato, and place onto each leaf.
- Wrap tightly.

TANTALIZING CHICKEN SALAD WITH BACON: RECIPE 14

Ingredients

- 1 large egg
- 4 oz. of chicken breast, skin and bone removed, sliced
- 1 cup of spinach, washed and dried

- 2 strips of bacon, cut into small pieces
- 1/4 of an avocado, peeled, seeded and diced
- 1 tablespoon of olive oil
- 1/2 a teaspoon of white vinegar
- salt and pepper, to taste

Instructions

- Boil the egg for 10 minutes in boiling water, then cool in cold water. Peel egg and then chop or slice.
- Heat a skillet over medium heat, add the chicken slices and cook for 3 minutes, or until cooked through.
- Move the chicken to the side and then add the bacon pieces, cook until your desired crispiness.
- In a mixing bowl, rip the spinach leaves then add the bacon, the chicken, and the chopped egg.
- Add the diced avocado, then drizzle with vinegar and olive oil.
- Season with salt and pepper, to taste.
- Toss together to coat all of the ingredients.
- Transfer to a serving plate.

GORGEOUS TUNA SALAD WITH AVOCADO: RECIPE 15

"Chicken works well here too, especially if you don't like tuna."

Ingredients

- 4 oz. can of tuna in brine or oil, drained
- 1 stalk of celery, diced
- 1/2 an avocado, peeled, seeded, and diced
- 2 tablespoons of mayonnaise
- 1 teaspoon of mustard
- 1/2 a teaspoon of fresh lemon juice

- salt and black pepper, to taste
- 1 egg, hard-boiled, peeled, and roughly chopped

Instructions

- In a mixing bowl, add the tuna, celery, and avocado.
- Add the mayonnaise, mustard, and the lemon juice.
- Add the egg to the tuna salad.
- Season with salt and black pepper.
- Mix well until combined.

CHICKEN-BROCCOLI CASSEROLE WITH CHEESE: RECIPE 16

Ingredients

- 10 oz. of chicken breast, skin and bone removed, sliced
- 2 cups of broccoli florets, fresh or frozen
- 2 tablespoons of olive oil
- 1/4 of a cup of sour cream
- 1/4 of a cup of heavy cream
- salt and black pepper, to taste
- 1/2 a teaspoon of oregano
- 1/2 a cup of cheddar cheese, grated
- 1 oz. of pork rinds, crushed

Instructions

- Preheat the oven to 230 degrees C.
- In a mixing bowl, add the chicken slices, broccoli, olive oil, and sour cream. Mix well to combine.
- Place mixture into a greased baking dish.
- Pour the heavy cream on top to cover the mixture and level it well.
- Season with salt and black pepper. Sprinkle with oregano.
- Sprinkle with grated cheddar cheese.
- Top with crushed pork rinds and bake for about 20-25

minutes, or until the chicken is cooked through.

YUMMY CHICKEN NOODLE SOUP: RECIPE 17

Ingredients

- 8 oz. of chicken breast, skin and bone removed, thinly sliced
- 2 tablespoons of olive oil
- 1/2 a white onion, chopped
- 1 medium carrot, peeled and chopped roughly.
- 2 stalks of celery, chopped into small pieces
- 1 tablespoon of dried oregano
- 1 quart of low-sodium chicken stock
- 1 large zucchini - spiralized
- a dash of sour cream

Instructions

- In a large skillet, heat olive oil over medium heat and cook the onion until tender.
- Add the chicken slices and cook until starting to brown on all sides.
- Add the carrots and celery. Add oregano and season with salt and black pepper. Cook until the carrots become soft.
- Add the low-sodium chicken stock and bring to a boil.
- Once boiled, lower the heat to a simmer.
- Add chicken pieces and cook for a further 20 minutes.
- Spiralize the zucchini into thin noodle strands. Add to the soup mixture in the last 2 or 3 minutes of it cooking.
- Transfer to serving dishes and add a dash of sour cream.
- Serve immediately.

AMAZING ASIAN BEEF AND COLESLAW: RECIPE 18

"One of my all-time favorite recipe!"

Ingredients

- 1 tablespoon of olive oil
- 2 cloves of garlic, crushed
- 1/2 a lb. of ground beef
- 5 oz. of coleslaw salad mix
- 1 tablespoon of low-sodium soy sauce
- salt and black pepper, to taste
- 1 teaspoon of sesame seeds
- 2 spring onions, chopped

Instructions

- In a wok or medium skillet, add a small amount of olive oil and heat over a medium-high heat.
- Heat the olive oil and add the crushed garlic. Cook until fragrant.
- Add the ground beef and brown until meat is cooked through, around 5 to 10 minutes. Stir while cooking and break up any lumps with a wooden spoon.
- When cooked, add in the coleslaw and stir to mix.
- Add in the olive oil and the low-sodium soy sauce.
- Stir and cook for around 5 minutes until the coleslaw mix starts to wilt.
- Season with salt and black pepper, to your taste.
- Serve with a sprinkle of sesame seeds and spring onion on the top.

CREAMY MUSTARD BEEF PATTIES: RECIPE 19

Ingredients

- 1 lb. of ground beef
- 1/2 a tablespoon of butter, unsalted
- 1 tablespoon of olive oil
- 1 spring onion, chopped finely
- 2 garlic cloves, minced or crushed finely
- 1/2 a cup of mushrooms, sliced thinly
- salt and black pepper, to taste

Mustard Cream Sauce

- 1/2 of a cup of heavy cream
- 1/2 a cup of white wine
- 2 tablespoons of Dijon mustard
- 1 large tomato, peeled and chopped
- 1 tablespoon of capers

Instructions

- Shape the beef into 6 patties and push your thumb in the center.
- Heat a large skillet over medium-high heat. Add the butter and melt until it begins foaming.
- Add the spring onion and garlic. Sauté until soft, for around 30 seconds.
- Season the beef patties with salt and black pepper. Cook until the desired degree of doneness is met. Turn once.
- Set to the side and keep warm.
- In the same skillet, add the mushrooms and sauté until limp. Add to the top of the warm patties.

To Prepare the Mustard Sauce:

- Deglaze the pan with the dry white wine. Cook and reduce the volume by half.
- Add the heavy cream and mustard followed by the tomato and capers.
- Heat slowly until hot (but do not boil).
- Pour the creamy mustard sauce over the beef patties and mushrooms.

CHEDDAR AND THYME PANCAKES: RECIPE 20

"Use any cheese that's your favorite!"

Ingredients

- 4 oz. of cheddar cheese, grated
- 2 egg yolks, beaten
- 1 teaspoon of butter
- 1/2 a cup of sour cream
- 1/2 a teaspoon of salt
- 1 teaspoon of thyme
- 1/4 of a teaspoon of dry mustard powder
- 1 tablespoon of protein powder, unflavored

Instructions

- In a mixing bowl, add the cheddar cheese with the sour cream and egg yolks, mix well together.
- In a small mixing bowl, add in the unflavored protein powder, fine salt, thyme, and dry mustard, mix well together.
- Add ingredients to a larger bowl and mix with the cheese and sour cream.
- Heat a medium skillet over medium heat, add the butter and melt.
- Add tablespoons of the batter to the skillet, maybe 3-4 at one time.

- Cook until lightly browned on the bottom and then flip and cook until golden brown on the second side.
- Serve immediately.

DELICIOUS CHICKEN SOUP WITH MUSHROOMS: RECIPE 21

Ingredients

- 1/2 a lb. of chicken breast, skin and bone removed, pound and thinly sliced
- 2 cups of low-sodium chicken stock
- 1 cup of fresh mushrooms, roughly chopped
- 4 tablespoons of sesame oil
- 2 tablespoons of sherry
- 2 tablespoons of fresh parsley, roughly chopped
- salt and black pepper, to taste

Instructions

- Thinly slice the chicken breasts into mouth-sized strips.
- In a medium pot, bring the chicken stock to a boil then add the chicken and mushrooms.
- When the soup begins boiling again, and all the ingredients float to the top, remove from the heat.
- Add the sesame oil and sherry, then stir and taste for seasoning.
- Add salt and black pepper, to taste.
- Spoon into individual soup bowls, and sprinkle the parsley on top.
- Serve immediately.

TERRIFIC TUNA BOATS WITH CUCUMBER: RECIPE 22

Ingredients

- 1 large cucumber
- 1 can of tuna in brine or oil, drained
- 1 egg, hardboiled, peeled, and diced
- 1/4 of a cup of cheddar cheese, grated
- 1 stick of celery, diced
- 2 tablespoons of mayonnaise
- 2 tablespoons of pickle relish
- 1 tablespoon of chopped green onion
- 1 teaspoon of fresh lemon juice
- 1/2 a teaspoon of salt

Instructions

- Cut the cucumber in half, and then slice into another two pieces.
- Remove the seeds with a small spoon. Run a peeler on the bottom side so they will sit flat.
- In a medium bowl, add all the remaining ingredients and combine.
- Spoon the mixture into the cucumber pieces.

BEAUTIFUL ASPARAGUS AND HAM BAKE: RECIPE 23

Ingredients

- 1/2 a lb. of cooked ham, chopped
- 3 oz. of cheddar cheese
- 2 tablespoons of butter, unsalted
- 1/4 of a cup of white onion, diced
- 1 cup of asparagus
- 3 large eggs
- 1/3 of a cup of heavy cream
- 1 teaspoon of dried mustard
- salt and black pepper, to taste

Instructions

- Preheat oven to 180 degrees C.
- In a large skillet over medium heat, add butter and once melted add the onion, ham and asparagus. Cook for around 3 minutes.
- In a medium mixing bowl, blend the eggs, cream, and the seasonings.
- Place the asparagus mixture in a medium baking dish, and then pour over the egg mixture. Bake for around 20 minutes.
- Sprinkle the top with grated cheese and then bake for an additional 10 minutes, or until cheese starts to brown.
- Divide between serving plates and eat while hot.

HASHED ZUCCHINI BROWNS: RECIPE 24

Kids like this one!

Ingredients

- 1 and a 1/2 lb. of zucchini
- 1/2 a teaspoon of salt
- 2 eggs
- 1/4 of a cup of parmesan cheese, grated
- 2 garlic cloves, pressed or minced
- 1/8 of a cup of butter, unsalted

Instructions

- Shred the zucchini coarsely to about 4 cups, into a medium bowl.
- Add salt and set aside, and let stand for 15 minutes.
- Squeeze the excess moisture with clean hands.
- Add the eggs, garlic, and cheese, then mix well to combine.
- In a large skillet over medium heat, heat 2 tablespoons of butter.

- Scoop about 2 tablespoons of the mixture together and then flatten in to form a patty, continue until all patties are formed.
- Add the patties to the skillet but avoid any overcrowding.
- Cook until golden on the bottom and then turn once. Continue to cook until golden, for around 6 to 8 minutes.
- Repeat with the remaining mixture until finished.
- Add more butter to the pan if needed.

FRITTATA WITH SAUSAGE: RECIPE 25

Ingredients

- 4 oz. of sausage, broken into small pieces
- 1/2 a green onion, chopped roughly
- 2 garlic cloves, minced or crushed
- 1/4 of a cup of ricotta
- 1/4 of a cup of heavy cream
- 2 eggs, beaten
- 1/4 of a teaspoon of cayenne pepper
- 1/8 of a cup of salsa
- 1/2 a cup of cheddar cheese, grated
- salt, to taste
- 1/4 of a cup of sour cream

Instructions

- Heat oven to 180 degrees C.
- In a skillet, sauté the onion and the garlic for around 30 to 40 seconds.
- Add broken up sausage pieces and cook until no pink remains.
- In a medium mixing bowl, add the heavy cream and the crumbled ricotta cheese.
- Add the beaten eggs, mixing with the salsa and the cayenne pepper.
- Pour over the sausage pieces in the skillet.

- Place the skillet in the oven and bake for 20 minutes, or until the frittata starts to firm up.
- Remove from oven and sprinkle with grated cheese.
- Place under a warmed broiler and cook until the cheese melts and becomes golden.
- Allow to cool a little then slice and serve with sour cream.

Chapter Five

KETOGENIC DINNER RECIPES

ZESTED ORANGE STIR-FRIED BEEF Recipe 26

"Great for entertaining!"

Ingredients

- 1/2 a lb. of beef steaks, sliced thinly
- 1/2 a cup of low-sodium beef broth
- 2 tablespoons of coconut oil
- 1 medium onion, diced
- 1/2 an orange, for zest and juice
- 4 cloves of garlic, minced or crushed
- 2 inches of sliced ginger
- a good pinch of ground cinnamon
- 1 teaspoon of low-sodium soy sauce
- 1/2 a teaspoon of fish sauce
- 1 bay leaf

Instructions

- Slice beef into 1-inch thin slices.

- Heat a medium skillet over medium-high heat and add coconut oil.
- Add the diced onion, garlic, and ginger, and sauté for 1 minute.
- Add the beef strips and cook for 5 minutes and add the soy sauce and fish sauce.
- Add the beef broth, bay leaf, cinnamon, and orange juice.
- Increase the heat and cook until broth juice has begun to thicken.
- Transfer to serving plates and top with orange zest. Serve hot.

SHRIMP WITH SWEET AND SPICY CHICKEN: RECIPE 27

Ingredients

- 2 chicken breasts, boneless and skinless
- 20 large shrimp, peeled
- 1/2 a cup of mushrooms, sliced
- 2 large handfuls of spinach
- 1/4 of a cup of mayonnaise
- 2 tablespoons of sriracha sauce
- 1 tablespoon of coconut oil
- 2 teaspoons of fresh lime juice
- salt and black pepper, to taste
- 1 teaspoon of garlic powder
- 1/2 a teaspoon of crushed red pepper
- 1/2 a teaspoon of paprika
- 1/2 a teaspoon of honey
- 1 spring onion, finely chopped

Instructions

- Tenderize chicken slices between plastic wrap until it is of a 1-inch thickness.
- Season with sea salt, black pepper, and garlic powder.
- In a skillet over medium heat, add the coconut oil and chicken breasts.

- Cook for 8 minutes and turn once. Reduce the heat and cover.
- Add the sliced mushrooms to the chicken. Add oil if required.
- In a mixing bowl, whisk together the mayonnaise, sriracha, and honey.
- Heat a pot over medium-high heat, and place the shrimp in one layer.
- Add the sauce and toss to coat. Cook for around 3 minutes until the shrimp are pink. Stir occasionally to prevent burning.
- Remove from the heat and add the fresh lime juice and toss to cover all the shrimp.
- Divide spinach onto serving plates with cooked mushrooms.
- Add the chicken and shrimp, and coat with the sauce.
- Sprinkle with chopped spring onion to garnish.

SPICY CHICKEN SLICE-UPS: RECIPE 28

"Jalapenos can go, if that's not your taste..."

Ingredients

- 2 tablespoons of olive oil
- 2 low-carb wraps
- 6 oz. of cheddar cheese, grated
- 2 chicken breasts, boneless and skinless, sliced into thin strips
- 1 avocado, peeled, pitted, and diced
- 2 teaspoons of chopped jalapenos
- 1/4 of a teaspoon of salt

Instructions

- In a skillet over medium heat, add a bit of oil and cook the chicken strips until browned and cooked through.

- In a large skillet, lay the wrap and warm over a medium heat. Heat for 2 minutes.
- Flip the wrap over and lay the grated cheddar cheese. Leave an inch of space close to the edges.
- Add the sliced chicken pieces, avocado, and jalapenos to half of the wrap.
- Fold the wrap over with a spatula and then press to flatten.
- The cheese sticks it together.
- Remove from the pan and cut into servable portions.

PERFECT SHRIMP WITH MUSHROOM NOODLES: RECIPE 29

Ingredients

- 20 large shrimp, peeled
- 16 oz. of mushrooms, sliced
- 1 tablespoon of olive oil
- 1 tablespoon of butter, unsalted
- 1 large zucchini
- 1 cup of marinara sauce
- salt and black pepper, to taste
- 2 tablespoons of parmesan cheese, grated

Instructions

- In a medium skillet over medium heat, add the olive oil.
- Fry the mushrooms until the oil has mostly been absorbed.
- Add butter to the skillet and cook for another 2 to 3 minutes.
- Add the shrimp and cook for around 4 minutes until they turn pink. Turn to avoid burning.
- Spiralize the zucchini to make the "noodles."
- Add the zucchini noodles to the cooked shrimp and toss. Cook for about 2 minutes while tossing.
- Pour the marinara sauce and season with salt and pepper.
- Cook until sauce is heated through.
- Transfer to serving plates and sprinkle with grated parmesan.

SPICED LIME STEAK AND ASPARAGUS: RECIPE 30

"This one is super-yummy!"

Ingredients

- 14 oz. of asparagus
- 1/2 a lb. of thin beef steak
- salt and black pepper, for seasoning
- olive oil, for cooking

Lime and Sriracha Sauce

- 1 lime, for juice
- 2 tablespoons of sriracha sauce, or more to taste
- 1/2 a teaspoon of vinegar
- salt and black pepper, to taste
- 1 tablespoon of olive oil

Instructions

- Place a medium skillet over medium-heat. Add a dash of olive oil.
- Fry the asparagus for around 10 minutes, toss to avoid burning.
- Season the steaks with salt and black pepper.
- Broil until cooked to your liking. Turn once.
- Remove from broiler and cover. Let the steak rest for 5 minutes.
- In a small mixing bowl, add the lime juice, vinegar and sriracha sauce. Add the salt and black pepper.
- Slowly pour the olive oil while whisking, to combine thoroughly.

- Slice the steaks into thin strips. Serve with fried asparagus and drizzle lime sauce over the top.

BEST BUNLESS BUTTER BURGER: RECIPE 31

Ingredients

- 1/2 a lb. of ground beef
- 2 tablespoons of butter, unsalted
- salt and black pepper, to season
- 2 cheese slices
- 2 teaspoons of mayonnaise
- 2 teaspoons of paprika
- 2 tablespoons of olive oil
- 2 lettuce leaves, washed and patted dry

Instructions

- In a small mixing bowl, season the ground beef with the salt, the pepper, and the paprika. Mix very well with clean hands.
- Form into 4 patties and place half of the butter in the center of 1 patty.
- Cover with the second patty, then press and seal the edges. Both patties will now be one.
- In a small skillet over medium-heat, add olive oil and cook the patties for 4 to 5 minutes on both sides.
- Flatten the lettuce leaves and spread with a little mayonnaise. Place a patty on the mayonnaise and top with the cheese slices.

GORGEOUS SEA BASS TOPPED WITH AVOCADO DRESSING: RECIPE 32

Ingredients

- 2 tablespoons of fresh lemon juice

- 2 tablespoons of fresh lemon zest
- 2 tablespoon of low-sodium soy sauce
- 2 teaspoons of Dijon mustard
- 2 medium-large sea bass fish fillets
- 1/2 a cup of pork rinds, crushed
- non-stick cooking spray

Sauce

- 1 medium avocado, peeled, pitted and coarsely chopped
- 1/2 of a cup of heavy cream
- 2 tablespoons of fresh lime juice
- 2 cloves of garlic, crushed or minced
- 2 dashes of hot sauce (optional)

Instructions

- Preheat oven to 230 degrees C.
- Add to a blender - the avocado, lime juice, heavy cream, garlic, and hot sauce, if using. Blend until you have a creamy mixture. Set aside.
- In a small mixing bowl, add the lemon juice, the lemon zest, the soy sauce, and the mustard.
- Dredge the fish fillets in the lemon juice mixture and coat with the crushed pork rinds.
- Spray non-stick spray onto a baking sheet.
- Place fish fillets on the baking sheet and cook in the oven for around 7 minutes. Turn once and cook for another 7 minutes, or until the fillets start to flake.
- Transfer to serving plates and drizzle with the avocado sauce.

CHEESY-TOPPED BAKED PORK: RECIPE 33

"Use chicken if you like!"

Ingredients

- 1/2 a lb. of pork steaks
- 3/4 of a cup of heavy cream
- 6 oz. of creamed cheese, cubed
- 1/4 of a cup of soy flour
- a pinch of salt and black pepper
- 1 teaspoon of paprika
- 1/2 a tablespoon of garlic salt
- 1/2 a cup of parmesan cheese, grated
- butter, for cooking

Instructions

- Slice pork steaks into thin strips.
- In a mixing bowl, combine the flour, salt, pepper, and the paprika.
- Coat the steak strips with the seasoned flour.
- Heat a skillet over medium-heat and add butter. When melted, cook the pork until brown on all sides.
- In a small pot, heat the cream and add the cream cheese, and then add the garlic salt with half of the parmesan cheese. Mix until well blended.
- Place pork pieces into the bottom of a small baking dish.
- Cover the strips with sauce, and with the remaining 1/4 of a cup of parmesan cheese sprinkled on the top.
- Bake for 20 minutes at 180 degrees C, or until golden brown.
- Divide between serving plates and serve hot.

SCRUMPTIOUS THREE-CHEESE PIZZA-QUICHE: RECIPE 34

Ingredients

- 1 cup of cheddar cheese, grated

- 1 oz. of cream cheese, softened
- 1 egg
- 1/8 of a cup of heavy cream
- 1/8 of a cup of parmesan cheese, grated
- 1/4 of a teaspoon of Italian seasoning
- 1/4 of a teaspoon of garlic powder
- 1/4 of a cup of pizza sauce, unsweetened
- 1/3 of a cup of mozzarella, torn into small pieces
- non-stick cooking spray

Instructions

- Preheat oven to 200 degrees C.
- In a mixing bowl, beat together the cream cheese, egg, parmesan cheese, and the spices.
- Spray a medium-sized, glass, baking dish with non-stick cooking spray.
- Add the cheddar cheese to the dish. Cover with egg mixture.
- Bake for around 20 to 30 minutes, or until the egg sets.
- Cover with pizza sauce and mozzarella cheese.
- Bake until browning and bubbly.
- Remove from oven and stand for 10 minutes before serving.

BEEF WITH STICKY SESAME SAUCE: RECIPE 35

"It's all about the sauce!"

Ingredients

- 1/2 a lb. of sirloin steak, cut into strips
- 2 tablespoons of honey
- 3 tablespoons of olive oil, divided into 2
- 2 tablespoons of low-sodium soy sauce
- 1/8 of a teaspoon of black pepper
- 2 spring onions, sliced thinly

- 2 garlic cloves, crushed or minced
- 1 tablespoon of sesame seeds
- 2 cups of brown rice, cooked

Instructions

- In a mixing bowl, add soy sauce, garlic, pepper, onions, honey, and sesame seeds. Mix until well combined.
- Add the beef strips to the bowl. Mix to coat with sauce and let sit for 15 to 20 minutes.
- In a skillet over high-heat, add 1 and a 1/2 tablespoons of olive oil.
- Add the beef strips and any juice, as well.
- Stir-fry until the beef browns, or to your desired taste.
- Serve warm over brown rice.

SOUTHWESTERN SIZZLING STEAKS: RECIPE 36

Cooking Mix

- 1/2 a lb. of beef steaks
- 2 cloves of garlic, crushed or minced
- 1/4 of a cup of white onion, roughly chopped
- 1/8 of a cup of green peppers, seeded and chopped
- 1/4 of a teaspoon of cumin powder
- 1/4 of a teaspoon of dried oregano

Marinade

- 2 tablespoons of dry white wine
- 1 teaspoon of olive oil
- 1/8 of a teaspoon of hot pepper sauce
- 1 tablespoon of low-sodium soy sauce
- 2 cloves of garlic, chopped or minced

Instructions

- In a mixing bowl, combine all the marinade ingredients and mix well.
- Add the steaks to the bowl. Coat steaks and then cover the bowl with plastic wrap. Refrigerate for 30 minutes or (ideally) overnight.
- Place a medium skillet over medium-heat. Add olive oil and sauté the onion, garlic, green peppers, oregano, and cumin for around 10 minutes.
- Taste and add garlic salt, if required.
- Remove steaks from refrigerator. Place in the skillet and cook for 5 minutes on both sides, or until cooked to your desired liking.
- Serve sizzling with your choice of sides.

SCRUMMY SAUSAGE PIE: RECIPE 37

"Use gourmet sausages for added flavor!"

Ingredients

- 8 oz. of sausage
- 8 oz. of cream cheese
- 2 eggs
- 1/3 of a cup of heavy cream
- 3 cups of zucchini, shredded
- 1/2 a cup of spring onions, roughly chopped
- salt and black pepper, to taste
- 3/4 of a cup of baking mix

Instructions

- Preheat oven to 205 degrees C.
- Preheat a medium skillet over medium-heat. Cook the sausage

in their own oil until no pink remains, and until they are
cooked all the way through.
- Mix well together with the baking mix, cream, and eggs.
- Arrange sausages in a spoke pattern in a medium baking dish.
- Pour baking mixture around the sausages in the baking dish.
- Add salt and pepper, to taste.
- Cook uncovered for around 30 minutes (or until starting to
  brown), and until the mixture is set.
- Serve immediately.

RECIPE#38: PAN-SEARED TOMATOES WITH STEAK AND EGGS

Ingredients

- 2 tablespoons of olive oil
- 1 lb. of thin beef steak
- 4 eggs
- 4 tomatoes, cut into halves
- salt and black pepper, to taste
- 1 tablespoon of fresh oregano, roughly chopped

Instructions

- Heat a large skillet over medium-high heat. Add 1 tablespoon
  of the olive oil.
- Season the steaks with salt and pepper on both sides and add
  to the skillet.
- Cook the steaks for about 4 to 5 minutes on each side.
- Remove steaks from skillet and let rest for 5 minutes. Cut into
  slices.
- Add the tomatoes cut-side down to the skillet, cook until
  browned for around 2 to 3 minutes.
- Add olive oil to the skillet and cook the eggs to your desired
  liking.
- Sprinkle the oregano over the tomatoes and eggs and season
  with salt and pepper, to taste.

- Serve warm with the steaks.

STIR-FRIED CHICKEN SAUSAGES: RECIPE 39

Ingredients

- 4 chicken sausages, sliced into bite-sized pieces
- 3 cups of broccoli florets, fresh or frozen
- 3 cups of spinach
- 1/2 of a cup of parmesan cheese, grated
- 1/2 of a cup of tomato Sauce
- 1/4 of a cup of red wine
- 2 tablespoons of butter, salted
- 2 cloves of garlic, minced or crushed
- 1/2 a teaspoon of red pepper flakes

Instructions

- Slice the chicken sausages into bite-sized chunks.
- In a medium saucepan, half fill with water and bring to a boil. Add the broccoli florets and cook for 5 minutes, or until tender.
- In a medium skillet over medium-heat, cook the sausage pieces until golden on all sides.
- Push the cooked sausage pieces to the side. Add the butter and melt.
- Add the garlic and sauté for 1 minute. Stir everything together and add the hot broccoli florets.
- Pour in the red wine and the pepper flakes, along with the tomato sauce.
- Combine everything and cook until heated.
- Add the spinach last.
- Season with the salt and pepper, to taste.
- Simmer for 5-10 minutes.

Chapter Six

KETOGENIC SNACK RECIPES

CRISPY-BAKED KALE CHIPS Recipe 40

"Kids love these!"

Ingredients

- kale leaves
- olive oil
- seasonings of choice

Instructions

- Preheat the oven to 190 degrees C.
- Wash and pat dry the kale leaves, thoroughly.
- Tear leaves into medium-sized pieces.
- Add to a large mixing bowl, a small amount of olive oil.
- Add kale leaves and spices.
- Mix with clean hands to coat all sides of the leaves.
- Place on baking sheet. Leave space in-between so air can pass through.
- Bake until crispy for around 8 to 10 minutes. Check at 2-minute intervals.

KETO ENERGY-BOOSTING PROTEIN SHAKE: RECIPE 41

Ingredients

- 1 and a 1/2 cup of almond milk
- 1 tablespoon of coconut oil
- 1 tablespoon of peanut butter
- 1 scoop of vanilla (or chocolate) protein powder
- 4 or 5 ice cubes

Instructions

- Add all the ingredients into a blender.
- Blend on high until you have a thick, creamy consistency.
- Pour and drink immediately, while cool.

SALTED ALMOND AND COCONUT BARK: RECIPE 42

Ingredients

- 1/2 a cup of almonds
- 1/2 a cup of flaked coconut, unsweetened
- 1 cup of dark chocolate, 70% cacao is great
- 1/2 a cup of coconut butter
- 1/4 of a teaspoon of sea salt
- 1 teaspoon of vanilla extract

Instructions

- Heat a skillet over medium-high heat, then add the almonds and coconut flakes. Roast for around 10 minutes, occasionally tossing to prevent burning.
- In a medium-sized double boiler, melt the chocolate. Once melted, add the coconut butter and vanilla extract. Mix well to combine.
- Remove and spread the mixture onto a lined baking sheet.

- Sprinkle the almonds and coconut flakes on the surface of the chocolate. Press the nuts down to sink into the chocolate.
- Sprinkle with a dash of salt and place in the refrigerator when cool.
- When thoroughly cooled, break into bite-sized pieces.

CHOCOLATE AND COCONUT CHEESECAKE: RECIPE 43

"A nice treat..."

Ingredients

Base

- 1/4 of a cup of almond meal
- 1/3 of a cup of shredded coconut, unsweetened
- 1-2 tablespoons of honey, to taste
- 2 tablespoons of melted butter, unsalted

Filling

- 1 cup of cream cheese, softened
- 6 tablespoons of coconut cream
- 2 tablespoons of cocoa powder
- 2 tablespoons of honey
- 2 teaspoons of coconut essence

Instructions

Base

- Preheat oven to 160 degrees C and lightly grease eight holes of a standard sized muffin tin (you can use non-stick spray if you wish).
- In a mixing bowl, add the almond meal, coconut, honey and the melted butter.

- Using clean hands, mix well until everything becomes combined.
- Divide the mixture into 8 portions and press into the muffin tin holes.
- Bake for 10 minutes, or until they turn golden brown.
- Remove from oven and let cool.

Filling

- In a mixing bowl, add all the ingredients for the filling.
- Using a hand mixer mix on low speed, blend until everything has combined.
- Once combined, increase speed to medium-high for 3 minutes.
- Spoon the mixture evenly between the cooled bases.
- Place in the refrigerator (before serving) for one hour.

CRISPY-BAKED PARSNIP CHIPS: RECIPE 44

Ingredients

- 2 medium parsnips, peeled and thinly sliced
- olive oil, for coating
- salt

Instructions

- Preheat oven to 190 degrees C.
- In a bowl, add the parsnip chips and drizzle with olive oil. Mix with clean hands and cover every side of the parsnip chips.
- Place on a lined baking sheet and leave space in-between chips.
- Bake for around 6 to 8 minutes, or until turning golden brown.
- Remove from oven and sprinkle with salt. Let cool before eating.

COCONUT-COVERED PEANUT BUTTER CHOCOLATE BALLS: RECIPE 45

"Peanut butter makes it so good!"

Ingredients

- 1/2 a cup of coconut oil
- 1/4 of a cup of grated coconut, unsweetened
- 1/4 of a cup of cocoa powder
- 4 tablespoons of peanut butter powder
- 6 tablespoons of hemp seeds, shelled
- 2 tablespoons of heavy cream
- 1 teaspoon of vanilla extract
- 30 drops of vanilla-flavored, liquid stevia

Instructions

- In a mixing bowl, add the dry ingredients. Mix well with a fork until combined.
- Add the coconut oil and knead until everything is combined and starts forming into a thick paste.
- Add the heavy cream, liquid stevia, and the vanilla. Mix again until everything is well-combined, and until you have a thick, creamy texture.
- Pour shredded coconut onto a plate.
- Form into balls using clean hands and roll in the grated coconut.
- Lay on a baking tray lined with parchment paper.
- Place in the freezer for around 30 minutes.
- Serve chilled.

YUMMY RASPBERRY AND LEMON ICE-POPS: RECIPE 46

Ingredients

- 6 popsicles
- 1 cup of raspberries, or other berries
- 1/2 a lemon, squeezed for the juice
- 1/4 of a cup of coconut oil
- 1 cup of coconut milk
- 1/4 of a cup of sour cream
- 1/4 of a cup of heavy cream
- 1/2 a teaspoon of guar gum
- 20 drops of liquid stevia

Instructions

- Add all ingredients to a mixing bowl. Blend the mixture with an electric blender.
- Blend on high speed until all the ingredients are mixed with the berries.
- Sieve the mixture to remove the seeds.
- Divide the mixture into popsicle molds and freeze until solid.
- Run the molds under hot water for a second or two to loosen the popsicles before consumption.

PERFECT PECAN AND MAPLE HEALTH BARS: RECIPE 47

"Kids love these so much!"

Ingredients

- 2 cups of pecan halves
- 1 cup of almond flour
- 1/2 a cup of golden flaxseed meal
- 1/2 a cup of grated coconut, unsweetened
- 1/2 a cup of coconut oil
- 1/4 of a cup of maple syrup
- 25 drops of liquid stevia

Instructions

- Preheat oven to 190 degrees C.
- Heat a skillet over medium-high heat. Add the pecan halves and cook for around 6 to 8 minutes.
- Remove from the skillet and stand to cool.
- Once cooled, place in a Ziploc bag and gently crush.
- In a mixing bowl, add the dry ingredients and mix with a fork to combine.
- Add the crushed pecans and combine them with the other ingredients.
- Add the liquid stevia, coconut oil, and the maple syrup. Mix well until a dough is formed. It will crumble a little.
- Push the dough into the base of a medium baking dish.
- Bake until the edges are starting to brown. Around 20-25 minutes.
- Remove from the oven.
- When partially cooled, place in the refrigerator for 1 hour.
- Cut into squares and remove with a spatula.

HONEY-KETO MUFFINS: RECIPE 48

Ingredients

- 1/2 a cup of blanched almond flour
- 1/2 a cup of flaxseed meal
- 1 tablespoon of psyllium husk powder
- 1/4 of a teaspoon of sea salt
- 1/4 of a teaspoon of baking powder
- 3 tablespoons of honey
- 1/4 of a cup of butter, melted
- 1 egg
- 1/3 of a cup of sour cream
- 1/4 of a cup of coconut milk
- 3 hot dogs

Instructions

- Preheat oven to 190 degrees C.
- In a large mixing bowl, mix the dry ingredients well.
- Add in the egg, butter, sour cream, and then mix well until combined.
- When everything is incorporated, add the coconut milk and continue mixing until you have a thick batter.
- Divide the batter between 20 greased muffin holes.
- Cut the hot dogs into 20 pieces and push a piece into each muffin hole.
- Bake for around 12 minutes. Put under the broiler for 1 to 3 minutes, or until the tops brown a little.

KETO MICROWAVED BROWNIES: RECIPE 49

Ingredients

- 1 tablespoon of creamy almond butter, unsalted
- 1 tablespoon of (beaten) egg white
- 1 teaspoon of cocoa powder, unsweetened
- 1/8 of a teaspoon of vanilla extract
- 3 drops of liquid stevia
- 1 pinch of baking soda
- 1 pinch of salt

Instructions

- Find a microwave-safe mug or container.
- In a small bowl, add the egg white and beat until they are aerated (nice and frothy).
- Place all ingredients in the mug and mix well with a fork.
- Microwave for about 40 seconds. You might have to experiment. Not all microwaves are equal in power setting functionality.
- For a "molten" consistency, knock off 10 seconds.

- Remove from microwave and top with maple syrup or cocoa powder.

JALAPENO POPPER BALLS: RECIPE 50

"A hint of hotness, great for a night with friends!"

Ingredients

- 3 oz. of cream cheese
- 3 slices of bacon
- 1 jalapeno pepper
- 1/2 a teaspoon of dried parsley
- 1/4 of a teaspoon of onion powder
- 1/4 of a teaspoon of garlic powder
- salt and black pepper, to taste

Instructions

- Place a medium-sized skillet over medium heat.
- Fry the bacon until very crispy.
- Once cooled, crumble.
- Remove the bacon and set onto one side. Keep the leftover grease for later use.
- Slice and de-seed the jalapeno pepper. Now, finely dice.
- In a mixing bowl, add the jalapeno and spices with the cream cheese and season with salt and pepper. Mix until well combined.
- Add the leftover bacon fat and mix until a solid ball has formed.
- Crumble the crispy bacon onto a plate.
- Divide the cream cheese mixture into 3 or 4 and then roll into balls with clean hands.
- Now roll the balls in the bacon bits to cover well.

IN CONCLUSION

Thank you so much for joining me here! I am so excited that you've decided to take your health into your own hands. It's always important to keep a positive mindset - and speaking from experience, I want you to know that some days will be harder than others. But hang in there, it gets easier over time.

Weight loss is definitely a journey with great reward. So, give yourself time to lose the weight you want, and make sure you are gentle on yourself. Make sure you have great people around you who will support, motivate, and inspire you. **Because you are totally worth it!** Sometimes all you need is a friend (or even a coach) to get you in the right frame of mind. I like to use meditation, yoga, gentle workouts, and nutrition as a solid base for myself. You can get some great tips online.

Just remember, no matter what you do, you always want to keep your safety and your overall health in the forefront of your mind. Because that's the end goal, isn't it? To be the best possible version of yourself that you can be. And I know you can do it, and you can add me to the list of people who support you, wholeheartedly.

I am always sending you my love and light in your weight loss and health journey. **Thank you for reading and making use of my book**.

Loads of love always, *Emma xx*

Please remember, if you haven't already read my mega title, "How I Lost 100 Pounds! My Personal Weight Loss Strategies for Optimum Happiness," make sure you get your FREE copy today. Inside you'll learn exactly how I lost my weight in 22 months, and the awesome benefits of knowing the right nutrition, and other amazing secrets including myths, water weight, cellulite prevention and removal, the only exercise you really need, the ancient and easy technique to help slim you quickly, how to balance meals, and much, much more! I hope you love it. It's my very special gift to you! Make sure you get your FREE copy today!

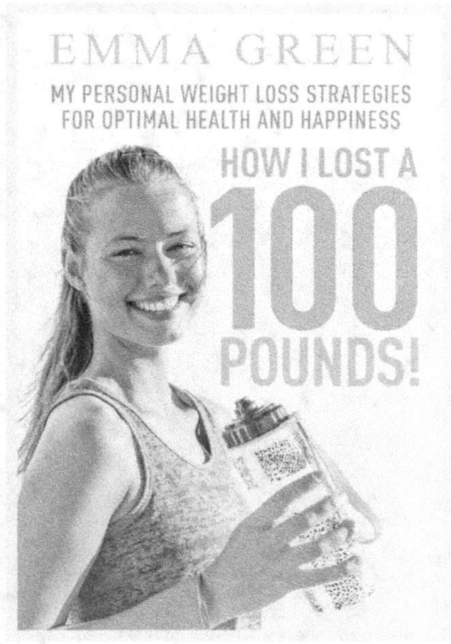

Click here for your FREE copy! xx